Diabetic Power Blends: *Energize and Thrive*

Healthy Eating

Table of Contents

Introduction

Welcome to "Diabetic Power Blends: Energize and Thrive," a one-of-a-kind smoothie recipe book specially crafted for individuals managing diabetes. This book is a celebration of the power of natural ingredients, blending together to create delicious and diabetic-friendly smoothies that nourish the body, balance blood sugar levels, and invigorate the spirit.

We understand that maintaining stable blood sugar levels is crucial for those with diabetes, and this book is designed with your needs in mind. Each smoothie recipe has been thoughtfully curated to include ingredients with a low glycemic index, focusing on whole foods that won't cause sharp spikes in blood sugar. By prioritizing nutrient-dense fruits, vegetables, and superfoods, we've crafted a collection of smoothies that not only taste divine but also contribute to your overall well-being.

In "Diabetic Power Blends: Energize and Thrive," you'll find an array of smoothies to suit different tastes and lifestyles. From delightful berry concoctions to creamy avocado blends and energizing green powerhouses, each recipe is a testament to the endless possibilities that lie within a blender. Whether you're starting your day with a nourishing breakfast or seeking a mid-day pick-me-up, these smoothies will keep you feeling energized and satisfied.

As you embark on this smoothie journey, know that the power to take charge of your health is in your hands. With these smoothie recipes, you'll discover the magic of blending nutrient-rich ingredients, creating tantalizing flavors, and managing your diabetes with a smile. Empower yourself with every sip as you enjoy a bounty of vitamins, minerals, and antioxidants in each glass.

In addition to the scrumptious recipes, we've included practical tips and insights to customize the smoothies to your taste and nutritional requirements. Feel free to experiment with ingredients, adjust sweetness to your preference, or incorporate protein sources that suit your dietary needs.

As you embrace the essence of "Diabetic Power Blends: Energize and Thrive," remember that nourishing your body is an act of self-care and love. Enjoy these smoothies mindfully, savoring every sip as you fuel your body and ignite your spirit with each delightful blend.

Here's to vibrant health, balanced blood sugar, and a journey of empowerment through the magic of smoothies. Get ready to energize and thrive, one sip at a time! Cheers to the power of blending and embracing a joyful and fulfilling life!

Recipe One: Green Power Smoothie

Ingredients:

- 1 cup fresh spinach or kale leaves, washed
- 1/2 ripe avocado, peeled and pitted
- 1/2 cucumber, peeled and chopped
- 1 cup unsweetened almond milk or coconut water
- 1 tablespoon chia seeds
- Ice cubes (optional, for a colder and thicker smoothie)

Instructions:

1. Prepare the Greens: Thoroughly wash the spinach or kale leaves to remove any dirt or debris. If using kale, remove the tough stems.
2. Prep the Avocado and Cucumber: Peel the ripe avocado and remove the pit. Use half of the avocado, saving the other half for another smoothie or dish. Peel and chop half of a cucumber into smaller pieces for easier blending.

3. Combine the Ingredients In a blender, add the washed greens, chopped avocado, chopped cucumber, and chia seeds.
4. Pour the Liquid: Pour in the unsweetened almond milk or coconut water into the blender. For a colder and thicker smoothie, add a few ice cubes as well.
5. Blend Until Smooth: Secure the blender lid and blend all the ingredients until smooth and creamy. If the mixture is too thick, add a bit more almond milk or water to reach your desired consistency.
6. Taste and Adjust: Taste the smoothie and adjust the flavor to your liking. If you prefer a sweeter smoothie, you can add a small amount of a low-calorie sweetener like stevia or a half teaspoon of honey (though this may slightly increase the sugar content).
7. Serve and Enjoy: Once the Green Power Smoothie reaches your desired consistency and taste, pour it into a glass. Optionally, you can garnish the smoothie with a sprinkle of chia seeds or a slice of cucumber. Enjoy the refreshing and

nutrient-packed smoothie immediately
while it's fresh and at its most nutritious!

The Green Power Smoothie is a vibrant and nourishing blend that packs a punch of essential nutrients, healthy fats, and hydration. With its earthy greens, creamy avocado, refreshing cucumber, and the superfood boost from chia seeds, this delightful concoction is a perfect choice to kickstart your day or recharge after a workout. Embrace the goodness of nature's power in every sip of this emerald elixir and let it fuel your body with vitality and strength. Cheers to a healthier you!

Recipe Two: Berry Delight Smoothie

Ingredients:

- 1 cup mixed berries (strawberries, blueberries, raspberries, or any combination)
- 1/2 cup plain Greek yogurt
- 1 tablespoon flaxseeds
- 1 cup unsweetened almond milk
- Ice cubes (optional, for a colder and thicker smoothie)

Instructions:

1. Select Your Berries: Choose a mix of your favorite berries or use a combination of strawberries, blueberries, and raspberries for a burst of flavor and antioxidants. Ensure the berries are fresh or frozen without added sugars.
2. Prep the Greek Yogurt: Measure half a cup of plain Greek yogurt, which is rich in protein and low in sugar compared to regular yogurt. It adds creaminess and tang to the smoothie.

3. Add Flaxseeds: Flaxseeds are a great source of fiber and healthy omega-3 fatty acids. Include one tablespoon of flaxseeds in the smoothie for added nutrition and a subtle nutty flavor.

4. Pour in Almond Milk: Measure one cup of unsweetened almond milk and add it to the blender. Almond milk complements the berries with its nutty taste and provides a dairy-free base.

5. Add Ice Cubes (Optional): For a refreshing and thicker smoothie, you can include a few ice cubes in the blender. It helps chill the smoothie and enhances its texture.

6. Blend Until Smooth: Secure the blender lid and blend all the ingredients until the mixture is smooth and the berries are fully incorporated. If you prefer a thinner consistency, you can add more almond milk.

7. Taste and Adjust: Take a moment to taste the smoothie. If you desire a sweeter flavor, you can add a touch of honey or a natural sweetener like stevia. However, keep in mind that the natural sweetness

from the berries and the creaminess from the yogurt might already be sufficient.

8. Serve and Enjoy: Pour the Berry Delight Smoothie into a glass and savor the delightful blend of berry goodness. Optionally, you can top it with a few fresh berries or a sprinkle of flaxseeds for an extra touch of elegance. Sip and enjoy the tangy and sweet symphony of berries with every refreshing sip!

The Berry Delight Smoothie is a delightful fusion of vibrant berries, protein-rich Greek yogurt, and nutty flaxseeds, all blended together with the smoothness of unsweetened almond milk. This refreshing concoction is not only a feast for the taste buds but also a nutritional powerhouse, brimming with antioxidants, fiber, and essential nutrients. Embrace the essence of these luscious berries and let this delightful smoothie become your go-to choice for a nourishing and satisfying treat any time of the day. Cheers to the joy of berries in a glass!

Recipe Three: Chocolate Banana Nut Smoothie

Ingredients:

- 1 ripe banana
- 1 tablespoon unsweetened cocoa powder
- 1/4 cup almonds or walnuts
- 1 cup unsweetened almond milk
- Ice cubes (optional, for a colder and thicker smoothie)

Instructions:

1. Prepare the Banana: Begin by peeling a ripe banana and cutting it into smaller chunks. Ripe bananas are sweeter and lend a creamier texture to the smoothie.
2. Add Unsweetened Cocoa Powder: Measure one tablespoon of unsweetened cocoa powder and add it to the blender. Cocoa powder brings in rich chocolate flavor without the added sugars.
3. Include Almonds or Walnuts: Choose between almonds or walnuts based on your preference, and add a quarter cup to

the other ingredients. Both nuts offer a dose of healthy fats, protein, and a nutty taste to the smoothie.

4. Pour in Almond Milk: Measure one cup of unsweetened almond milk and add it to the blender. The almond milk will provide a smooth and nutty base for the smoothie, perfectly complementing the flavors of chocolate and banana.

5. Add Ice Cubes (Optional): If you desire a colder and thicker smoothie, include a few ice cubes in the blender.

6. Blend Until Smooth: Secure the blender lid and blend all the ingredients until the mixture turns smooth and creamy. The combination of chocolate, banana, and nuts will create a delectable and indulgent flavor profile.

7. Taste and Adjust: Take a moment to taste the Chocolate Banana Nut Smoothie. If you prefer a sweeter taste, you can add a small amount of honey or a natural sweetener, but keep in mind that the natural sweetness from the ripe banana might already be sufficient.

8. Serve and Enjoy: Pour the Chocolate
    Banana Nut Smoothie into a glass.
    Optionally, you can sprinkle a pinch of
    cocoa powder or crushed nuts on top for
    an extra chocolatey or nutty touch. Sip
    and revel in the delightful blend of
    chocolate, banana, and nutty goodness!

The Chocolate Banana Nut Smoothie is a decadent fusion of rich chocolate, creamy banana, and the nutty goodness of almonds or walnuts. Each sip is a blissful indulgence, reminiscent of a luscious chocolate dessert. This smoothie is perfect for satisfying your chocolate cravings or as a nourishing post-workout treat. Embrace the delightful flavors of chocolate and banana in a glass and let the Chocolate Banana Nut Smoothie become your guilt-free pleasure for a moment of sweet satisfaction! Cheers to the heavenly combination of chocolate and bananas!

Recipe Four: Cinnamon Apple Spice Smoothie

Ingredients:

- 1 medium-sized green apple, cored and chopped
- 1/2 cup plain Greek yogurt
- 1/2 teaspoon ground cinnamon
- 1 tablespoon almond butter
- 1 cup unsweetened almond milk
- Ice cubes (optional, for a colder and thicker smoothie)

Instructions:

1. Prep the Green Apple: Start by washing the green apple thoroughly to remove any dirt or residue. Core the apple and chop it into smaller pieces, ensuring it's ready to blend smoothly.
2. Measure the Greek Yogurt: Scoop half a cup of plain Greek yogurt into a measuring cup. Greek yogurt adds creaminess and a dose of protein to the smoothie.

3. Add Ground Cinnamon: Sprinkle half a teaspoon of ground cinnamon into the measuring cup with the Greek yogurt. Cinnamon not only enhances the flavor but also adds a warm, comforting spice to the smoothie.

4. Include Almond Butter: Add one tablespoon of almond butter to the other ingredients. Almond butter brings in healthy fats, protein, and a nutty taste, complementing the apple-cinnamon combination.

5. Pour in Almond Milk: Measure one cup of unsweetened almond milk and add it to the blender. The almond milk serves as the liquid base for the smoothie, and its subtle nuttiness pairs well with the other ingredients.

6. Add Ice Cubes (Optional): If you prefer a colder and thicker smoothie, include a few ice cubes in the blender.

7. Blend Until Smooth: Secure the blender lid and blend all the ingredients until the mixture turns smooth and creamy. The green apple will release its tangy sweetness, harmonizing with the

comforting flavors of cinnamon and
almond butter.

8. Taste and Adjust: Take a moment to taste
   the Cinnamon Apple Spice Smoothie. If
   you desire a sweeter taste, consider adding
   a small amount of honey or a natural
   sweetener, but keep in mind the natural
   sweetness from the apple and cinnamon
   might be sufficient.

9. Serve and Enjoy: Pour the Cinnamon
   Apple Spice Smoothie into a glass.
   Optionally, you can sprinkle a pinch of
   ground cinnamon on top for a delightful
   aroma and added visual appeal. Sip and
   indulge in the warm and cozy blend of
   apple and spice, as the flavors dance on
   your palate with each sip!

The Cinnamon Apple Spice Smoothie is a
delightful fusion of tangy green apple, warm
cinnamon, creamy almond butter, and protein-
rich Greek yogurt. With every sip, you'll be
transported to a cozy fall day, wrapped in the
comforting embrace of apple pie spices. This
smoothie is perfect for chilly mornings or as an
afternoon treat to lift your spirits and tantalize

your taste buds. Embrace the joy of apple spice in a glass and let the Cinnamon Apple Spice Smoothie become your go-to indulgence for a touch of seasonal magic any time of the year! Cheers to the heartwarming flavors of apple and spice!

Recipe Five: Tropical Paradise Smoothie

Ingredients:

- 1 cup ripe mango, peeled and diced
- 1 cup fresh pineapple, peeled and diced
- 1/2 cup coconut milk (unsweetened)
- 1 tablespoon fresh lime juice
- Fresh mint leaves (a few leaves for garnish, optional)
- Ice cubes (optional, for a colder and thicker smoothie)

Instructions:

1. Prep the Mango and Pineapple: Begin by peeling a ripe mango and cutting it into small, juicy chunks. Do the same with the fresh pineapple, removing the outer skin and core, and dicing it into bite-sized pieces. Make sure to use ripe fruits to enhance the natural sweetness of the smoothie.
2. Measure the Coconut Milk: Pour half a cup of unsweetened coconut milk into a measuring cup. Coconut milk adds a

creamy and tropical flavor to the smoothie while keeping it dairy-free.

3. Squeeze Fresh Lime Juice: Cut a fresh lime in half and squeeze the juice into the measuring cup with the coconut milk. The tangy lime juice will balance the sweetness of the tropical fruits.

4. Add the Fruits and Liquid: In a blender, combine the diced mango and pineapple with the coconut milk and lime juice. For a colder and thicker smoothie, you can include a few ice cubes as well.

5. Blend Until Smooth: Secure the blender lid and blend all the ingredients until the mixture becomes smooth and creamy. The vibrant colors of the mango and pineapple will blend harmoniously, creating a tropical oasis in your glass.

6. Garnish with Fresh Mint (Optional): If you desire an extra burst of freshness, add a few fresh mint leaves to the blender. Mint complements the tropical flavors and elevates the experience of sipping the smoothie.

7. Taste and Adjust: Take a moment to taste the Tropical Paradise Smoothie. If needed,

you can adjust the sweetness or tartness by adding a touch of honey or more lime juice, depending on your preference.

8. Serve and Enjoy: Pour the Tropical Paradise Smoothie into a glass, and if you included mint leaves, they will add a beautiful touch as a garnish. Sip and revel in the taste of a tropical paradise, with the exotic blend of mango, pineapple, coconut, and lime transporting you to a blissful island getaway!

The Tropical Paradise Smoothie is a heavenly fusion of ripe mango, fresh pineapple, creamy coconut milk, and zesty lime. With every sip, you'll embark on a journey to a faraway tropical island, where the sun-kissed fruits dance on your taste buds. It's a delightful treat that captures the essence of a beach vacation in a single glass. Whether you enjoy it as a refreshing breakfast or a rejuvenating afternoon pick-me-up, this Tropical Paradise Smoothie is sure to add a splash of sunshine and pure bliss to your day! Cheers to a taste of the tropics!

Recipe Six: Creamy Berry Avocado Smoothie

Ingredients:

- 1 cup mixed berries (strawberries, blueberries, raspberries, or any combination)
- 1/2 ripe avocado
- 1/2 cup plain Greek yogurt
- 1 tablespoon flaxseeds
- 1 cup unsweetened almond milk
- Ice cubes (optional, for a colder and thicker smoothie)

Instructions:

1. Select Your Berries: Choose a mix of your favorite berries or use a combination of strawberries, blueberries, and raspberries for a burst of flavor and antioxidants. Ensure the berries are fresh or frozen without added sugars.
2. Prep the Avocado: Cut the ripe avocado in half and remove the pit. Scoop out half of the avocado flesh and add it to the blender. Save the other half for another

smoothie or use it in salads or other
dishes.

3. Measure the Greek Yogurt: Scoop half a cup of plain Greek yogurt into the blender. Greek yogurt adds creaminess and a boost of protein to the smoothie.

4. Add Flaxseeds: Include one tablespoon of flaxseeds in the blender. Flaxseeds are a great source of fiber and healthy omega-3 fatty acids, adding an extra nutritional punch to the smoothie.

5. Pour in Almond Milk: Measure one cup of unsweetened almond milk and add it to the blender. Almond milk serves as the liquid base for the smoothie, providing a dairy-free option and a subtle nutty flavor.

6. Add Ice Cubes (Optional): For a colder and thicker smoothie, you can include a few ice cubes in the blender.

7. Blend Until Smooth: Secure the blender lid and blend all the ingredients until the mixture becomes smooth and creamy. The creamy avocado will meld with the sweet-tart berries, creating a luscious and velvety texture.

8. Taste and Adjust: Take a moment to taste the Creamy Berry Avocado Smoothie. If desired, you can add a touch of honey or a natural sweetener to enhance the sweetness, but keep in mind the natural sugars from the berries might already be sufficient.

9. Serve and Enjoy: Pour the Creamy Berry Avocado Smoothie into a glass and enjoy the delightful blend of creamy avocado and mixed berries. Optionally, you can top the smoothie with a few extra berries or a sprinkle of flaxseeds for added texture and presentation. Sip and savor the smoothie's creamy goodness, packed with a medley of flavors and nutrients!

The Creamy Berry Avocado Smoothie is a delicious fusion of creamy avocado, vibrant mixed berries, and protein-rich Greek yogurt. With each sip, you'll be treated to a velvety smoothie that combines the creaminess of avocado with the burst of berry sweetness. This nutrient-packed delight is perfect for a refreshing breakfast, a post-workout treat, or a guilt-free dessert. Embrace the creaminess of avocado and the tanginess of mixed berries in a glass, and let the Creamy Berry Avocado Smoothie become your go-to indulgence for a dose of wholesome goodness! Cheers to the creamy and berrylicious blend!

Recipe Seven: Citrus Splash Smoothie

Ingredients:

- 2 oranges or tangerines (peeled and segmented)
- 1 large carrot (peeled and chopped)
- 1-inch piece of fresh ginger (peeled and grated)
- 1/2 teaspoon ground turmeric
- 1 cup unsweetened coconut water or water
- Ice cubes (optional, for a colder and thicker smoothie)

Instructions:

1. Prepare the Citrus Fruits: Peel the oranges or tangerines and separate them into segments, removing any seeds or pith. Freshly squeezed orange or tangerine juice works as well if you prefer not to use segments.
2. Chop the Carrot: Peel the large carrot and chop it into smaller pieces for easier blending. Carrots add natural sweetness and a boost of nutrients to the smoothie.

3. Grate the Fresh Ginger: Use a grater to grate a 1-inch piece of fresh ginger. Ginger adds a zesty kick and anti-inflammatory properties to the smoothie.

4. Add Ground Turmeric: Sprinkle half a teaspoon of ground turmeric into the blender. Turmeric not only adds a vibrant golden color but also brings its anti-inflammatory benefits.

5. Pour in Coconut Water or Water: Measure one cup of unsweetened coconut water or water and add it to the blender. Coconut water adds a tropical twist and hydration, while water provides a neutral base.

6. Add Ice Cubes (Optional): If you prefer a colder and thicker smoothie, include a few ice cubes in the blender.

7. Blend Until Smooth: Secure the blender lid and blend all the ingredients until the mixture becomes smooth and well combined. The citrusy and gingery aromas will invigorate your senses.

8. Taste and Adjust: Take a moment to taste the Citrus Splash Smoothie. If you desire a sweeter taste, consider adding a small amount of honey or a natural sweetener,

but keep in mind that the natural
sweetness from the citrus fruits and
carrots might be enough.

9. Serve and Enjoy: Pour the Citrus Splash
   Smoothie into a glass. Optionally, you can
   garnish the smoothie with a slice of
   orange or a sprinkle of ground turmeric
   for a visually appealing touch. Sip and
   revel in the refreshing and zesty blend of
   citrus fruits and ginger with every
   delightful sip!

The Citrus Splash Smoothie is a refreshing
fusion of juicy citrus fruits, vibrant carrots, zesty
ginger, and the subtle warmth of turmeric. With
every sip, you'll experience a burst of tangy
flavors, balanced with the earthy notes of ginger
and turmeric. This invigorating and nutrient-rich
blend is perfect for starting your day with a
revitalizing kick or as a hydrating treat after a
workout. Embrace the zesty splendor of citrus
and ginger in a glass and let the Citrus Splash
Smoothie become your go-to elixir for a
refreshing and nourishing pick-me-up! Cheers to
the invigorating citrusy splash!

Recipe Eight: Minty Cucumber Lime Smoothie

Ingredients:

- 1 medium cucumber (peeled and chopped)
- Juice of 1 lime
- A handful of fresh mint leaves
- 1 cup baby spinach (optional, for extra greens)
- 1 cup unsweetened coconut water or water
- Ice cubes (optional, for a colder and thicker smoothie)

Instructions:

1. Prepare the Cucumber: Start by peeling the medium cucumber to remove any tough skin. Chop the cucumber into smaller pieces for easier blending.
2. Extract Lime Juice: Squeeze the juice of one lime into a measuring cup or bowl. Freshly squeezed lime juice adds a zesty and tangy twist to the smoothie.
3. Include Fresh Mint Leaves: Take a handful of fresh mint leaves and add them

to the blender. Mint leaves provide a refreshing and cool flavor to the smoothie.

4. Add Baby Spinach (Optional): If you desire additional greens, you can include one cup of baby spinach in the blender. Spinach adds nutrients and enhances the vibrant green color of the smoothie.

5. Pour in Coconut Water or Water: Measure one cup of unsweetened coconut water or water and add it to the blender. Coconut water brings a tropical touch and hydration, while water provides a neutral base.

6. Add Ice Cubes (Optional): For a colder and thicker smoothie, you can include a few ice cubes in the blender.

7. Blend Until Smooth: Secure the blender lid and blend all the ingredients until the mixture becomes smooth and well combined. The invigorating scents of mint and lime will awaken your senses.

8. Taste and Adjust: Take a moment to taste the Minty Cucumber Lime Smoothie. If you desire a sweeter taste, consider adding a small amount of honey or a natural sweetener, but keep in mind that the

natural freshness of cucumber and lime might be sufficient.

9. Serve and Enjoy: Pour the Minty Cucumber Lime Smoothie into a glass. Optionally, you can garnish the smoothie with a sprig of fresh mint or a slice of cucumber for a delightful visual touch. Sip and relish in the cooling and refreshing blend of mint, cucumber, and lime with every invigorating sip!

The Minty Cucumber Lime Smoothie is a rejuvenating blend of crisp cucumber, zesty lime, and fresh mint leaves. With each sip, you'll experience a burst of cooling flavors, making it an ideal choice for a hot summer day or a revitalizing morning drink. This hydrating and nutrient-packed smoothie is perfect for energizing your body and refreshing your mind. Embrace the invigorating combination of mint, cucumber, and lime in a glass, and let the Minty Cucumber Lime Smoothie become your go-to elixir for a refreshing and revitalizing sip any time you need a little pick-me-up! Cheers to the minty-citrus delight!

Recipe Nine: Nutty Banana Spinach Smoothie

Ingredients:

- 1 ripe banana
- 1 cup baby spinach leaves
- 1 tablespoon almond butter or peanut butter (natural, no added sugar)
- 1 cup unsweetened almond milk or any milk of your choice
- 1/2 teaspoon ground cinnamon (optional, for added flavor)
- Ice cubes (optional, for a colder and thicker smoothie)

Instructions:

1. Prepare the Banana: Start by peeling a ripe banana and cutting it into smaller chunks. Using ripe bananas adds natural sweetness to the smoothie.
2. Add Baby Spinach: Take one cup of baby spinach leaves and add them to the blender. Spinach adds a dose of nutrients and vibrant green color to the smoothie.

3. Include Nut Butter: Choose between almond butter or peanut butter based on your preference, and add one tablespoon to the blender. Both nut butters provide healthy fats and a nutty flavor to the smoothie.

4. Pour in Almond Milk: Measure one cup of unsweetened almond milk or any milk of your choice and add it to the blender. Almond milk serves as the liquid base for the smoothie and complements the nutty flavors.

5. Add Ground Cinnamon (Optional): For an extra burst of flavor, sprinkle half a teaspoon of ground cinnamon into the blender. Cinnamon pairs well with banana and nut butter.

6. Add Ice Cubes (Optional): If you prefer a colder and thicker smoothie, include a few ice cubes in the blender.

7. Blend Until Smooth: Secure the blender lid and blend all the ingredients until the mixture becomes smooth and creamy. The combination of banana, nut butter, and spinach creates a delightful and nutritious blend.

8. Taste and Adjust: Take a moment to taste the Nutty Banana Spinach Smoothie. If desired, you can add more cinnamon for a stronger cinnamon flavor or a touch of honey for extra sweetness.

9. Serve and Enjoy: Pour the Nutty Banana Spinach Smoothie into a glass. Optionally, you can garnish the smoothie with a sprinkle of ground cinnamon or a slice of banana for an appealing touch. Sip and enjoy the creamy and nutty goodness, with the delightful blend of banana and spinach adding a nutritious twist to your day!

The Nutty Banana Spinach Smoothie is a creamy and nutty blend of ripe banana, nutritious spinach, and the richness of almond or peanut butter. With each sip, you'll experience the delightful combination of sweet banana and nutty goodness, all wrapped in the goodness of spinach. This smoothie is a wholesome and satisfying choice for breakfast or a post-workout refuel. Embrace the creaminess of banana and nut butter with the nourishment of spinach in a glass, and let the Nutty Banana Spinach

Smoothie become your go-to elixir for a
flavorful and nourishing start to your day!
Cheers to the nutty-banana green delight!

Recipe Ten: Peanut Butter and Jelly Smoothie

Ingredients:

- 1 cup frozen mixed berries (strawberries, blueberries, raspberries)
- 2 tablespoons creamy peanut butter (natural, no added sugar)
- 1 cup unsweetened almond milk or any milk of your choice
- 1 tablespoon chia seeds
- 1 tablespoon honey or maple syrup (optional, for added sweetness)
- Ice cubes (optional, for a colder and thicker smoothie)

Instructions:

1. Prepare the Frozen Berries: Measure one cup of frozen mixed berries. You can use a combination of strawberries, blueberries, and raspberries, or choose your favorite berries. Using frozen berries adds a refreshing and chilled element to the smoothie.

2. Add Creamy Peanut Butter: Scoop two tablespoons of creamy peanut butter into the blender. Make sure to use natural peanut butter without any added sugars or oils.

3. Include Chia Seeds: Add one tablespoon of chia seeds to the other ingredients. Chia seeds offer a dose of healthy omega-3 fatty acids and create a thicker texture in the smoothie.

4. Pour in Almond Milk: Measure one cup of unsweetened almond milk or any milk of your choice and add it to the blender. Almond milk serves as the liquid base and pairs well with peanut butter and berries.

5. Add Honey or Maple Syrup (Optional): If you desire a sweeter taste, you can include one tablespoon of honey or maple syrup. However, keep in mind that the natural sweetness from the berries and peanut butter might already be sufficient.

6. Add Ice Cubes (Optional): For a colder and thicker smoothie, include a few ice cubes in the blender.

7. Blend Until Smooth: Secure the blender lid and blend all the ingredients until the

mixture turns smooth and creamy. The combination of peanut butter and berries will create the classic Peanut Butter and Jelly flavor.

8. Taste and Adjust: Take a moment to taste the Peanut Butter and Jelly Smoothie. If desired, you can add more honey or maple syrup for extra sweetness or adjust the thickness by adding more almond milk or ice cubes.

9. Serve and Enjoy: Pour the Peanut Butter and Jelly Smoothie into a glass. Optionally, you can garnish the smoothie with a sprinkle of chia seeds or a berry on top for a visually appealing touch. Sip and relish the classic peanut butter and jelly goodness in a nutritious and flavorful blend!

The Peanut Butter and Jelly Smoothie is a delightful blend of creamy peanut butter and sweet mixed berries, reminiscent of the classic childhood sandwich. With each sip, you'll experience the nostalgic taste of peanut butter and jelly, all while enjoying a nutritious and satisfying smoothie. This smoothie is perfect for breakfast or a quick snack that will satisfy your taste buds and keep you energized throughout the day. Embrace the familiar and comforting flavors of peanut butter and jelly in a glass, and let the Peanut Butter and Jelly Smoothie become your go-to treat for a wholesome and enjoyable experience! Cheers to the peanut butter and jelly goodness!

Recipe Eleven: Tropical Green Smoothie

Ingredients:

- 1 cup fresh spinach leaves
- 1/2 ripe banana
- 1/2 cup fresh or frozen pineapple chunks
- 1/2 cup fresh or frozen mango chunks
- 1/2 cup unsweetened coconut water or coconut milk
- 1 tablespoon chia seeds (optional, for added nutrients)
- Ice cubes (optional, for a colder and thicker smoothie)

Instructions:

1. Prepare the Fresh Spinach: Start by washing the fresh spinach leaves thoroughly to remove any dirt or debris. Fresh spinach provides a nutritious and vibrant green base for the smoothie.
2. Prep the Banana: Peel a ripe banana and cut it into smaller chunks. Ripe bananas

add natural sweetness and creaminess to
the smoothie.

3. Add Pineapple and Mango: Use fresh or
   frozen pineapple and mango chunks. Both
   fruits bring in tropical flavors and natural
   sweetness to the smoothie.

4. Pour in Coconut Water or Coconut Milk:
   Measure half a cup of unsweetened
   coconut water or coconut milk and add it
   to the blender. Coconut water or milk
   complements the tropical fruits and
   provides a delightful island flavor.

5. Include Chia Seeds (Optional): If you
   desire added nutrients and a thicker
   texture, add one tablespoon of chia seeds
   to the blender. Chia seeds offer fiber,
   healthy fats, and a protein boost.

6. Add Ice Cubes (Optional): For a colder
   and thicker smoothie, you can include a
   few ice cubes in the blender.

7. Blend Until Smooth: Secure the blender
   lid and blend all the ingredients until the
   mixture becomes smooth and creamy. The
   combination of spinach, banana,
   pineapple, and mango creates a refreshing
   and tropical blend.

8. Taste and Adjust: Take a moment to taste
    the Tropical Green Smoothie. If needed,
    you can add a touch of honey or a natural
    sweetener to enhance the sweetness, but
    keep in mind that the natural sugars from
    the fruits might already be sufficient.
9. Serve and Enjoy: Pour the Tropical Green
    Smoothie into a glass. Optionally, you can
    garnish the smoothie with a slice of
    pineapple or a sprinkle of chia seeds for
    added texture and presentation. Sip and
    savor the tropical goodness, as the fresh
    flavors transport you to a sunny beach
    destination with each delightful sip!

The Tropical Green Smoothie is a refreshing and
nourishing blend of fresh spinach, sweet
pineapple, creamy mango, and the tropical touch
of coconut. With every sip, you'll be transported
to a paradise of flavors and vibrant colors. This
tropical delight is perfect for brightening up your
mornings or as a revitalizing afternoon treat.
Embrace the tropical vibes and the nourishment
of greens in a glass, and let the Tropical Green
Smoothie become your go-to elixir for a taste of

paradise any time you need a little getaway! Cheers to the tropical green indulgence!

Recipe Ten: Chocolate Almond Chia Smoothie

Ingredients:

- 1 cup unsweetened almond milk
- 1 tablespoon almond butter (natural, no added sugar)
- 1 tablespoon chia seeds
- 1 tablespoon unsweetened cocoa powder
- 1 ripe banana
- 1/2 teaspoon vanilla extract
- Ice cubes (optional, for a colder and thicker smoothie)

Instructions:

1. Prepare the Almond Milk: Measure one cup of unsweetened almond milk and add it to the blender. Almond milk serves as the smoothie's liquid base and complements the almond butter.
2. Add Almond Butter: Scoop one tablespoon of almond butter into the

blender. Ensure that the almond butter is natural without any added sugars or oils.

3. Include Chia Seeds: Add one tablespoon of chia seeds to the other ingredients. Chia seeds will add a nutritional boost and create a thicker consistency in the smoothie.

4. Mix in Unsweetened Cocoa Powder: Add one tablespoon of unsweetened cocoa powder to the blender. Cocoa powder will bring a rich and chocolatey flavor to the smoothie without any added sugars.

5. Prep the Ripe Banana: Peel a ripe banana and add it to the blender. Ripe bananas provide natural sweetness and contribute to the smoothie's creamy texture.

6. Add Vanilla Extract: Include half a teaspoon of vanilla extract to enhance the overall flavor of the smoothie.

7. Add Ice Cubes (Optional): For a colder and thicker smoothie, you can include a few ice cubes in the blender.

8. Blend Until Smooth: Secure the blender lid and blend all the ingredients until the mixture turns smooth and creamy. The combination of chocolate and almonds

will create a delectable and indulgent flavor profile.

9. Taste and Adjust: Take a moment to taste the Chocolate Almond Chia Smoothie. If desired, you can add more cocoa powder for a richer chocolate flavor or adjust the sweetness by adding a small amount of honey or maple syrup.

10. Serve and Enjoy: Pour the Chocolate Almond Chia Smoothie into a glass. Optionally, you can sprinkle a pinch of cocoa powder or a few chia seeds on top for added texture and presentation. Sip and relish the delightful blend of chocolate and almond goodness with every luscious sip!

The Chocolate Almond Chia Smoothie is a luxurious and nutty blend of almond butter, rich cocoa, and the nutritious goodness of chia seeds. With each sip, you'll experience a burst of chocolatey indulgence with the subtle nutty undertones of almonds. This smoothie is perfect for satisfying your chocolate cravings or as a nourishing post-workout treat. Embrace the delectable combination of chocolate and almonds in a glass, and let the Chocolate Almond Chia Smoothie become your go-to elixir for a moment of sweet satisfaction! Cheers to the chocolatey and nutty delight!

Recipe Twelve: Veggie Power Smoothie

Ingredients:

- 1 cup fresh spinach leaves
- 1/2 cucumber (peeled and chopped)
- 1 medium carrot (peeled and chopped)
- 1/2 ripe avocado
- 1/2 lemon (juiced)
- 1 tablespoon fresh ginger (peeled and grated)
- 1 cup unsweetened coconut water or water
- A few ice cubes (optional, for a colder and thicker smoothie)

Instructions:

1. Prepare the Fresh Spinach: Begin by washing the fresh spinach leaves thoroughly to remove any dirt or debris. Fresh spinach provides a nutritious and vibrant green base for the smoothie.
2. Prep the Cucumber and Carrot: Peel the cucumber and carrot to remove any tough skin. Chop the cucumber and carrot into smaller pieces for easier blending.

3. Scoop the Avocado: Cut a ripe avocado in half, remove the pit, and scoop out half of the avocado flesh. Save the other half for another smoothie or use it in salads or other dishes.
4. Squeeze Lemon Juice: Juice half of a lemon to extract its zesty and tangy juice. The lemon juice will add brightness and balance to the smoothie.
5. Grate Fresh Ginger: Use a grater to grate one tablespoon of fresh ginger. Ginger adds a zesty kick and anti-inflammatory properties to the smoothie.
6. Pour in Coconut Water or Water: Measure one cup of unsweetened coconut water or water and add it to the blender. Coconut water provides hydration and a subtle tropical touch, while water serves as a neutral base.
7. Add Ice Cubes (Optional): If you prefer a colder and thicker smoothie, include a few ice cubes in the blender.
8. Blend Until Smooth: Secure the blender lid and blend all the ingredients until the mixture becomes smooth and well combined. The combination of spinach,

cucumber, carrot, and avocado creates a nourishing and refreshing blend.

9. Taste and Adjust: Take a moment to taste the Veggie Power Smoothie. If desired, you can add a pinch of salt or a small amount of honey to enhance the flavors to your liking.

10. Serve and Enjoy: Pour the Veggie Power Smoothie into a glass. Optionally, you can garnish the smoothie with a cucumber slice or a sprinkle of grated ginger for added texture and presentation. Sip and embrace the power of veggies in a glass, as you enjoy the nutritious and invigorating taste with every delightful sip!

The Veggie Power Smoothie is a nutritious and vibrant blend of fresh spinach, cucumber, carrot, creamy avocado, zesty lemon, and zingy ginger. With each sip, you'll experience a burst of nourishing goodness and the invigorating flavors of the garden's finest. This smoothie is perfect for kickstarting your day with a boost of vegetables or as a refreshing pick-me-up any time you need an energy boost. Embrace the power of veggies in a glass and let the Veggie Power Smoothie become your go-to elixir for a wholesome and revitalizing experience! Cheers to the veggie-filled vitality!

Recipe Thirteen: Pineapple Cucumber Mint Splash Smoothie

Ingredients:

- 1 cup fresh pineapple chunks
- 1/2 cucumber (peeled and chopped)
- A handful of fresh mint leaves
- 1 cup unsweetened coconut water
- Ice cubes (optional, for a colder and thicker smoothie)

Instructions:

1. Prepare the Fresh Pineapple: Start by cutting fresh pineapple into chunks. If you prefer a colder smoothie, you can use frozen pineapple chunks instead.
2. Prep the Cucumber: Peel the cucumber to remove any tough skin, and chop it into smaller pieces for easier blending. Using a cucumber adds a refreshing and hydrating element to the smoothie.
3. Include Fresh Mint Leaves: Take a handful of fresh mint leaves and add them

to the blender. Mint leaves provide a refreshing and cool flavor to the smoothie.

4. Pour in Coconut Water: Measure one cup of unsweetened coconut water and add it to the blender. Coconut water adds a tropical twist and natural sweetness to the smoothie.

5. Add Ice Cubes (Optional): For a colder and thicker smoothie, include a few ice cubes in the blender.

6. Blend Until Smooth: Secure the blender lid and blend all the ingredients until the mixture becomes smooth and well combined. The tropical flavors of pineapple and the coolness of cucumber will blend with the refreshing essence of mint.

7. Taste and Adjust: Take a moment to taste the Pineapple Cucumber Mint Splash Smoothie. If desired, you can add a small amount of honey or a natural sweetener to enhance the sweetness, but keep in mind that the natural sugars from the pineapple might already be sufficient.

8. Serve and Enjoy: Pour the Pineapple Cucumber Mint Splash Smoothie into a

glass. Optionally, you can garnish the smoothie with a mint sprig or a slice of cucumber for an appealing touch. Sip and savor the tropical and refreshing blend, as the combination of pineapple, cucumber, and mint transports you to a sunny beach destination with every delightful sip!

The Pineapple Cucumber Mint Splash Smoothie is a refreshing and hydrating blend of tropical pineapple, cooling cucumber, and the delightful essence of mint. With each sip, you'll experience a burst of refreshing flavors, making it an ideal choice for a hot summer day or a revitalizing morning drink. This smoothie is perfect for energizing your body and refreshing your mind. Embrace the tropical vibes and the cooling sensation in a glass, and let the Pineapple Cucumber Mint Splash Smoothie become your go-to elixir for a refreshing and revitalizing sip any time you need a little pick-me-up! Cheers to the pineapple-cucumber-mint delight!